MW00843449

WORK SMARTER, NOT HARDER

A Nurse's Guide to Managing and Prioritizing Patient Care

WORK SMARTER, NOT HARDER

A Nurse's Guide to Managing and Prioritizing Patient Care

Written by Joann Coleman

Copyright © 2020, Joann Coleman. All rights reserved.

This book or any portion thereof may not be reproduced or used in any manner whatsoever without the publisher's express written permission except for the use of brief quotations in a book review.

Printed in the United States of America

First Printing, 2020

ISBN13: 978-1-951883-07-2

The Butterfly Typeface Publishing
PO Box 56193
Little Rock AR 72215

www.thebutterflytypeface.com

"With the love of nursing and prayer, I share this book with you in hopes that like me, you too will have an amazing journey."

Joann Coleman

"Nursing is an art of the heart."

TABLE OF CONTENTS

FOREWORD

Working Smarter, Not Harder: A Nurse's Guide to Managing and Prioritizing Patient Care will serve as a guided platform for nurses from all experience levels (whether novice or highly seasoned) to provide safe and effective care to patients in all areas of nursing specialty.

According to the Bureau of Labor Statistics' Employment Projections, Registered Nursing (RN) is among the top occupations in terms of job growth through 2026.

The RN workforce is expected to grow from 2.9 million in 2016 to 3.4 million in 2026, an increase of 438,100 or 15%. The Bureau also projects the need for an additional 203,700 new RNs each year through 2026 to fill newly created positions and to replace nurses (American Association of Colleges of Nursing (AACN/Nursing Shortage Fact Sheet).

With these alarming statistics, our profession will demand that nurses are qualified with professional and interpersonal skills.

Disease burden resulting from unhealthy lifestyle choices such as smoking, excessive alcohol use, drugs, physical inactivity, and stress will no doubt cause the health care system to become even more overloaded. This doesn't even include acute and chronic illnesses such as diabetes, heart disease, cancer, kidney disease, and not to mention the overwhelming uprising of infectious diseases.

The statistics are alarming! Therefore, it is imperative that nurses create and continue to work smart, not hard on behaviors that will promote safe patient outcomes and be involved in facilitating a workplace environment that is conducive for diversity and learning.

I will share my experience with you in hopes of paving the way for you to develop your own path to a successful career in nursing.

While I talk a lot about working smart, not hard, I will also reinforce throughout this book that *Work Smarter, Not Harder*, isn't the green light to take shortcuts on practices and policies that have been established and governed by the State Board of Nursing, including the Nurse Practice Act and your employment organization.

My goal is to share my years of nursing experience and knowledge to provide tidbits of information regarding my journey from being that nervous new graduate to the "seasoned" nursing professional I am today.

Again, no matter where you are in terms of your experience level, this book will help guide you with insightful, helpful, and humorous ways to work smart, not hard.

I pray that it will help you to avoid some of the pitfalls I've made in my career.

Joann Coleman/Author

ACKNOWLEDGMENTS

With heartfelt gratitude and thanks to the millions of nurses who have dedicated their lives to helping others, this book is dedicated to you! Your value is unsurmountable! Through challenges, you remained resilient, through challenges, you remained ready, and through challenges, you remained. I also want to give a heartfelt thanks to my family for your continued love, support, and encouragement throughout this amazing journey. Most importantly, I thank God for giving me the opportunity to share words of wisdom now and throughout my nursing career.

INTRODUCTION

As I began my journey writing this book, much like being a new nurse, I was very anxious. But I was reminded of Philippians 4:6-7:

"Do not be anxious about anything, but in everything by prayer and petition, with thanksgiving, present your request to God. And the peace of God, which transcends all understanding, will guard your hearts and minds in Christ Jesus."

So, as you begin your journey into nursing (and even if you're seasoned like me), be reminded of this scripture when you're afraid, nervous, or unsure.

Nursing has made tremendous strides for improvements since I graduated from nursing school in 1984.

I'd like to refer to those days as the "horse and buggy days of nursing." Professional practices, supported by evidence-based outcomes, has grown by leaps and bounds. Gone are the days of shakedown mercury thermometers, hand-counting narcotics from a photo album-like book stuffed with what seemed like hundreds of pills and ampules.

Among other things, computerized charting and bar code medication administration are just a few of the changes that have made our career easier in terms of time while providing means for safer patient outcomes.

Technological advancements, along with specialized training, preceptorship programs, and mentoring (just to name a few), have catapulted the "horse and buggy days of nursing" into the *nowadays* of a profession that is continually evolving and is "second to none!"

No matter what educational level you've achieved or level of experience you've attained thus far, by the end of this book, you will agree that nursing really begins in the heart.

CHAPTER ONE
Love What You Do

First, to be smart, love what you do!

My journey began while caring for my mother. Mom was diagnosed with multiple sclerosis in the early 1970s. I watched and cared for her (along with five younger brothers and sisters) as she suffered from a disease that was not recognized during this time.

Through all her sufferings, she subsequently passed away at the young age of 36, leaving behind seven children: my twin sister (seventeen and seniors in high school) and five other children whose ages ranged from three to eleven.

The loss of my mother was very tragic for all of us, although my younger siblings have only vague to no memories of her. In my opinion, that was a good thing for them because for me, remembering the many nights of severe seizure-like spasms, the complete blindness, countless ambulance calls and visits to the emergency room, and extended inpatient hospital stays were torture.

Caring for my mom was one thing but seeing how she was treated was also impactful. I didn't know it then, but God was preparing me for my calling while I rendered care to my mom to the best of my young ability.

I can recall one visit in particular as if it were yesterday.

I was with my mother in a Chicago hospital. At that time, the Multiple Sclerosis was advanced. She was completely blind and had a tracheostomy, an opening surgically created through the neck into the windpipe to allow for breathing. During this time, the tracheostomy was plugged to allow her to talk, eat certain foods, and take medications.

"Mrs. Greene, my name is Ms. Littles. I'm your nurse, and it's time for your pills," the young female nurse who was probably in her 30's said to my mother in a sterile manner and shoved the cup of pills into my mother's weak hands.

Because my mother was blind and could not see what or how many pills were in the medication cup, my mother accidentally spilled some of the pills onto the floor.

"What's wrong with you!?" The nurse screamed at my mother, angrily, "Can't you hold a cup of pills!?"

"No," my mother answered flatly, "I'm blind."

Helpless, as the tears streamed down my face, I was frozen in shock and disbelief as I witnessed someone speaking to a person in that tone who was totally dependent on them for care.

That memory is still etched in my mind, and I'm often reminded of that memory as I render care to my patients. I'm also reminded of the words from Maya Angelou, "It's not what people say, but how they make you feel." This quote helps me to guard my heart and exercise control over the things that come out of my mouth. I'll be the first to say it can be very difficult when managing difficult patients, family members, and coworkers, but I have learned throughout my journey that our words really do have the power to hurt or heal.

That experience taught me an invaluable lesson: When you love what you do, you don't have to work hard at it.

Probably like nursing today, that young nurse was rushing to complete her tasks, but she missed the opportunity to administer her greatest task, which is to offer love and care to her patient, something that is not found in a pill.

Nursing pays a very lucrative salary in comparison to a lot of other professions. It also offers the ability to work overtime, to travel, to moonlight in positions that can pay you just as much (or more) as your primary job and affords you to work for as long as you desire. I have never been unemployed in the last 30+ years.

While the earning potential is great, if you don't love what you do, it will manifest itself in behaviors similar to the painful one my mother encountered.

I cannot emphasize this enough.

Loving what you do is exhibited by your work ethics and the interactions you have with your patients, their families, coworkers, and physicians.

When you love what you do, you don't have to work hard at it.

Consider this:

What were your personal reasons for choosing nursing as a career? Do you love what you do? Why? Why not?

_____

_____

_____

_____

_____

_____

_____

_____

_____

_____

_____

CHAPTER TWO
Dare to Be Different

Be smart! Be different!

Dare to be different is another piece of advice based on my journey to *Work Smarter, Not Harder* that I'd like to share with you. Be prepared to meet resistance and sometimes isolation when being different. Some people may not like or understand that your standards decide for you to not gossip or participate in behaviors that are not conducive to a healthy work environment.

Please understand me when I say that it's perfectly okay to be involved in fun activities at work. Distance yourself from people who are not ready to share work ethics that promote workplace safety and cohesiveness. Unprofessional conduct like gossiping, rumor-mongering are starters for toxic environments, so avoid these situations by not being the lighter fluid to create these fires. Avoid these situations by being different!

Now, don't get me wrong. We work long hours, and I am one who enjoys communication, laughter, and most of all, potlucks. Even in the Bible, Ecclesiastes Chapter 13 clearly spells it out, "There is a time and place for all things under the Heavens." Please understand that I don't advocate being in jail and not having any get out of jail free cards. I do believe in balance in the workplace.

Always strive to maintain a level of professionalism in the workplace. Situations can get out of hand very quickly when someone feels intimidated or feel they have been treated unfairly. Sometimes tension rises due to misunderstandings. For example, a nurse may feel she or he has been given an unfair assignment.

Communication is the key to maintaining professionalism in the workplace. Always remember that everyone reacts and responds differently when being confronted about a situation. When dealing with a difficult situation, try to understand what happened and listen carefully to both sides of the story without being opinionated or taking sides. Being different means being a good listener.

Dare to be different by not engaging in unethical behavior, including statements or remarks and bouts of anger on social media. This is huge! I know several nurses who have been fired because of comments made in anger on social media that cannot be recanted, removed, or renounced. Once you hit send, it's out there for the world to make its judgment on you and your character. The verdict can be costly! *Work smarter, Not harder* by being different.

Dare to be different by being a mentor or preceptor to a new graduate nurse. The reality of graduating from nursing school, passing the state boards, and practicing as a new nurse can be a real shock for a new graduate nurse.

I believe wholeheartedly it is during this time that new nurses formulate their perception of their new careers, and it is at this point where they can be molded to become the professional nurses that are needed in the profession.

Transitioning into practice rests heavily on us as experienced nurses. That is why it is so important to maintain a level of professional behavior and work ethics.

New nurses mimic the behaviors of those around them. New graduate nurses have achieved the theoretical foundation of nursing, but they are now being faced with the professional responsibilities that are not within their grasp at this early phase of their careers.

Simply put, they are not practice-ready. However, with mentoring, guidance, and time, they can and will become the professional nurses that are desperately needed.

There is a stigma in nursing that states, "Nurses eat their young."

Dare to be different by not being a part of devouring and destroying the confidence that new nurses need.

Feelings of professional isolation and horizontal violence (discussed in a later chapter) are just a few issues that new graduates feel.

Consider this:

What are you doing today, or what can you change today to dare to be different?

_____

_____

_____

_____

_____

_____

_____

_____

_____

_____

_____

_____

Work Smarter, Not Harder

_____

_____

_____

_____

_____

_____

_____

_____

_____

_____

_____

_____

_____

CHAPTER THREE
Learn All You Can

Third, to be smart, learn all you can!

Learn all you can and then some. This is the third rule of learning how to *Work Smarter, Not Harder*. I can recall shortly after graduating from nursing school. I didn't pass my state boards the first time. Talk about heartbreaking; I cried for days while my other friends went about their careers as new RNs. Again, I believe that in every experience and every situation God places you in, there are valuable lessons to be learned. So, as I began to accept the reality of not passing my boards the first time, I feel strongly today that it was a lack of preparation on my part. As I was so excited to have graduated, I was shocked back into reality after realizing I had not put in the required time to study for state boards.

Once I understood the seriousness of my actions, I began to take time out to study and prepare. I felt as though I were the only one who had ever failed the boards, but after some time, I found out there were others in my class and previous classes who hadn't passed as well.

Some classmates had to retake boards as many as three times, while others gave up.

The feelings of disappointment and hurt, along with shame, were just some of the feelings I internalized during this time. Don't allow yourself to linger in these feelings if you experience not passing state boards the first time. It is natural to feel this way after having worked so hard in school.

Don't give up!

After you've identified your areas of weakness, begin to concentrate and study hard. Not passing state boards does not affect your success in nursing. In fact, I know a nurse who failed the boards three times and became (and still is) one of the best Neonatal Intensive Care Unit (NICU) nurses in the United States.

Fortunately, I passed the second time around. I was so excited to have passed. Now I would not have to drive to Little Rock, Arkansas, test for two days, and wait for weeks to get my results. My how times have changed!

My first job after passing the state boards was in a very small rural hospital in my hometown of Marianna, Arkansas. The small rural hospital setting was just what I needed as a new graduate starting out. The small hospital had an emergency room, labor and delivery, medical-surgical, and pediatrics all under one roof. It was time to put into action all that I had learned in theory and clinical throughout nursing school.

I had an excellent group of instructors in nursing school, each with their different personalities but very serious about the business of molding and modeling behaviors that produced prudent and competent nurses.

As a matter of fact, I can still hear my instructor saying, "Are you sure?" as I practice to this very day.

My instructors were firm on the teachings of principles in nursing. Principles in nursing are constant. They will never change. There are principles in nursing including treating every individual with respect, dignity, and compassion, and owning and taking responsibility for your actions that are aligned with the professional bodies of nursing law. These are just a few of the nursing principles that were instilled in me as a young nurse.

Practices in nursing have and will continue to change, but principles will never change. Nursing principles are the very foundation of what constitutes safe patient outcomes based on effective nursing care.

"Ding. Ding. Ding."

It was the sound of the emergency room doorbell. It was dark and was probably around 8:30 pm. The doors stayed locked after dark because it was a small rural hospital. We knew it was serious because whoever was ringing the bell was pressing it continuously. I was in training as a new nurse, and my preceptor, "Rena," was a highly trained ER nurse who could run a "Code Blue" with one eye closed.

I absolutely admired her and looked up to her as being one of the smartest nurses I had ever known. She was a real mentor to me.

We opened the door to the ER, and there stood a gentleman in an obvious state of panic. He looked like he'd seen a ghost.

"My…my…my…w…w…w..wife is in labor," he stuttered.

We could hear his heavy breathing. We weren't sure who needed help – him or his wife. Her voice was screaming like a siren. Rena and I gazed at each other and realized what was about to happen.

I ran out of the Emergency Room door with a wheelchair to assist the young woman. She was in the 4th quarter of labor, and the clock was ticking. Of course, I had never delivered a baby. I'd only observed a delivery once in nursing school, and since practicing as a nurse, I've never been a Labor and Delivery Nurse (L&D), and after that night, I have no desire to be one.

I pushed the wheelchair with care and speed with the young woman screaming violently. My preceptor and I got her onto an exam table in the ER, and this is when the fun (or not so fun) part began.

"This is how you learn," my preceptor said to me as she handed me an OB kit and slammed the door to the exam room.

"Bam."

Although I have never been in jail, I can relate the sound of Rena closing that door to that of someone being locked up in jail. Nowhere to go, this is it. Reality settled in.

"Ahhhhhh!!!" the soon mother-to-be screamed at the top of her lungs.

I screamed too, "Rena. I need help!"

But Rena had stepped out of hearing range. Although I was a brand-new nurse, and it never occurred to me to press the little red emergency button on the wall to summon for help. I was scared to death. I couldn't believe Rena had left me alone in this situation.

While I know now that Rena only wanted to provide a learning platform for me, I also realize that was a very unsafe practice, one that could have led to very serious consequences, including litigation and loss of license.

Labor and Delivery is one of the highest liability areas of nursing practice, highly unpredictable, with two lives at stake.

Not knowing the woman's history made this situation a very dangerous one as well. As the baby's head began to crown, I saw thick, curly black hair, and although I was nervous, I felt excited too. My adrenaline was what kept me standing on my feet.

As the baby started to descend further, I noticed that the baby's color was not very good, ashy like not pink like I was accustomed to seeing new babies look like.

The mother continued to push as her maternal instincts allowed her to do so. My hands were trembling, and I was sweating, just like the mother was. I noticed that the umbilical cord was wrapped around the baby's neck not once, but twice (known as a double nuchal cord).

I know God was with me and that mother on this night.

"Stop pushing," I said calmly to the mother. I didn't want to alarm her.

I eased one or two of my shaking fingers under the nuchal cords and slipped them around the little baby's head one at a time.

The baby made a full descent, and I could see it was a boy.

I started smacking him on his bottom like he had done something to me! Next, I heard the sweetest sound; he made a strong cry.

His color returned to the nice pink color that I remembered newborn babies looked like, and he began to breath normally. It seemed like an eternity, but all of that happened very quickly. I hadn't had time to panic.

I dried, wrapped, and placed the baby on his mother's tummy. Luckily, the husband had come around, but then, I fainted. The next thing I knew, I was being aroused by some type of aroma that Rena was wafting under my nose.

Consider this:

What are you doing to stay knowledgeable in your field of expertise?

CHAPTER FOUR
Mentoring and Preceptorship

For new graduates, it is vital for their success to engage in mentoring through a good preceptorship program. It is important for them not to be tossed out into the deep water without a life jacket, similar to the experience I encountered with Rena.

Real growth into your new role can be established during this time. In contrast, without good preceptorship during this time, it can have a negative impact on your growth. It doesn't necessarily mean you can't still experience growth, but it can delay growth and potentially cause you to rethink your career decision.

Your preceptor will be your shadow for the specific time frame that your facility has outlined for your orientation. Your orientation is tailored to meet your individual needs and goals as outlined by your employment facility.

One of the roles of a nursing preceptor is to mentor and educate you during the orientation process. During the "horse and buggy" days of nursing, there were no formal mentoring or preceptor programs, nursing education departments, or nurse educators like today. You were thrown into the deep water, and you had to back float, dog paddle, or do whatever in order to survive.

We did the best with the resources that were available to us at the time.

Preceptors assigned to new nurses help to establish goals based on facility policy and procedures, skills checklists, and clinical competencies.

Maintaining professionalism while keeping the lines of communication open between you and your preceptor will ensure your success at the beginning of your journey.

An effective preceptor communicates expectations, answers questions clearly, allows an opportunity for feedback and explains the reason and rationale for decisions.

I have had the opportunity to serve as a nursing preceptor at various hospitals during my nursing career, and it has given me great joy to see young nurses grow into their full potential professionally and personally.

There are five key factors to ensure you are teamed up with a good preceptor:

1. Make sure your preceptor can be a good listener and can easily identify when you may not understand something.
2. Make sure your preceptor has acquired knowledge and expertise that you will surely need.
3. Does your preceptor have a passion and a sincere desire to mentor?
4. Will your preceptor be willing to take you to the next level by challenging you to raise the standards for yourself?
5. Is your preceptor a positive role model?

Make it a point and a priority to learn as much as you can during your orientation process with your preceptor. As a matter of fact, learn all you can along your nursing journey. Knowledge is the key to staying abreast of the trends in nursing.

At the age of 60 and during the writing of this book, I made the decision to return to school to obtain my bachelor's degree in Nursing (BSN). It was important for my professional growth to make this decision, one that I should have made earlier, but life happened. It is also a testament to you that it's never too late to obtain knowledge. I encourage you to continue your educational journey.

The small rural hospital where I began my career can't measure up to the larger hospitals where I've been employed that have libraries on site and programs within the facility that offer opportunities for growth in education.

Although I am proud of my humble beginnings, I'm just simply making a comparison to the availability and access to knowledge.

Information in a few seconds is now available through the internet with literally millions of websites that offer teaching tools, simulations, webinars, etc.

Get curious. Offer to observe a procedure on your unit. Ask questions, and don't be afraid to communicate. Ask questions from physicians, surgeons, and other specialty physicians in your facility.

I've found that most doctors love to teach and welcome questions.

Most medication administration computers have access to tools such as Microdex and Mosby's. With just a click, you can obtain knowledge regarding a particular medication, dosages, side effects, etc. Access to these links provides learning opportunities and education for the patient, family members, and you.

As I mentioned, knowledge is key. Continuing education is important during your journey to becoming a successful nurse.

Cardiology was my first love, as I've had the opportunity to work alongside many cardiologists, including electrophysiologists and interventional cardiologists. Moreover, the knowledge I've gained has and will remain an important part of my nursing journey.

Although in some hospital settings, there are telemetry or monitor techs who are responsible for analyzing cardiac rhythms, I still to this day will take a patient's monitor strip and measure the intervals and the rhythm because of my love of cardiology and learning. Assume the responsibility of self-learning by learning a new skill set. Concentrate and practice until you've perfected it. Take advantage of all the learning opportunities your hospital offers outside of those that are required.

Technology offers a wealth of learning opportunities; however, refuse to allow technology to eliminate the benefit of hands-on learning.

Nursing school is mainly theory-based. The real learning comes when you begin to practice as a licensed nurse.

Love to learn. This is another piece of advice to working smarter!

Consider this:

Are you willing to become a mentor? What new learning opportunities have you acquired? What goals have you set for yourself to advance your knowledge or education?

CHAPTER FIVE
The Nurse Practice Act

During nursing school, become familiar with your state's Nurse Practice Act. This knowledge serves as a guide and governs nursing practices for each state in which you may practice. This is an important area of knowledge for working smarter:

Every nurse (not just a few) is responsible for knowing the state's Nurse Practice Act for the jurisdiction in which he or she holds a license.

Being accountable and responsible for the standards and scope of nursing practice is critical to your success as a nurse. Visit your state board of nursing website to gain insightful information regarding the board's mission, licensure, statues, rules, etc.

Working Smarter, Not Harder includes knowing your Nurse Practice Act; after all, not knowing is not an excuse for not being prepared for the consequences of your actions as it pertains to the professional code of conduct for nurses.

Beyond a shadow of a doubt, when we wake up every morning and prepare ourselves to go to our places of employment, none of us have the intention to hurt or harm any patient who is under our care. But again, to *Work Smarter, Not Harder*, you must be prepared by knowing your Nurse Practice Act, your job responsibilities, and the responsibilities of those who are assuming care under your jurisdiction, such as LPNs, nursing assistants, etc.

I experienced a "near-miss" incident along my journey that I can share as it relates to knowing the responsibilities of other nurses under your jurisdiction.

A "near-miss" is an unplanned event that does not result in injury, illness, or damage, but has the potential to do so.

I can recall working a hectic 3-11 pm shift. I was the charge nurse this particular day. The LPN had been assigned to a patient who was post-PTCA

(Percutaneous Transluminal Coronary Arthroplasty). Post PTCA cardiologists almost always infuse the drug Integrilin (platelet aggravator). The beginning of the shift, as always, was crazy busy – phones jumping off the hook, admissions arriving, discharges, someone bleeding profusely, etc. You name it; we had it that day.

The pump started alarming in Room 307. The Integrilin had almost infused, but the patient had to receive another dose. Again, this was in the "horse and buggy" days of nursing.

The LPN assigned to Mr. Jones, in Room 307, informed me that the medication (Integrilin) was almost completed and asked if she could go to the pharmacist to pick up the next dose.

"Yes," I said, thankful that she was eager to help and volunteer to walk to the pharmacy since I was too busy to pick up the last dose of Integrilin. Upon her return from the pharmacy, she noticed that I was very busy. She asked if it was ok for her to hang the Integrilin.

Being so busy and distracted, I said, "Yes, you can hang the Integrilin."

She was an excellent LPN, and I would trust her with my life. She was comparable to some of the best RNs with whom I'd ever worked. She was very thorough, knowledgeable, and skilled. I learned from some of the best "old school" LPNs in Memphis. LPNs who were charge nurses in the ICU took me under their wings, and I learned from them.

So, she hung the Integrilin.

The bottle of Integrilin was 100ml to infuse over 10 hours, which meant it was to infuse at 10cc/hour.

When I heard the infusion pump alarm in one hour, I knew right away what had happened, although I prayed like never before that it wasn't what I thought.

When I entered the room, my suspicion was correct. The bottle of Integrilin that should have infused over 10 hours had infused in one hour. The pump had been set to infuse at 100cc/hour instead of 10cc/hour.

I stood there in disbelief. All the noise and commotion around me silenced while I said to myself, "I can't believe this is happening."

Everything that had been so important was not so important now.

A lot of times, we get too busy and caught up in things that take away our attention from the task at hand. Most importantly, my attention was now on the patient to ensure his safety. Profuse bleeding and development of a hematoma at the puncture site were all serious concerns, a retroperitoneal bleed! For nurses, it's like we have a checklist of things to complete with only so many hours to complete them in. The clock is always racing in our minds. Also, the checklist does not include any unexpected occurrences such as an unexpected fall, adjustments in staffing due to a coworker becoming ill at work, and suddenly has to leave; the list of unexpected occurrences goes on and on.

Oh, my God.

I checked the patient's groin and vital signs and attempted to pull myself together as I tried to prepare my speech to a very intense, no-nonsense interventional cardiologist. I immediately called him after gathering my assessment and vital signs and explain to him exactly what happened.

Extra monitoring was required.

I cried and prayed. I prayed and cried. But I had to keep my composure as the shift had to continue to run.

Again, God sent angels to protect the patient, the LPN, and me. Fortunately, the relatively young patient had very few co-morbidities, and blessings were on our side. Understandably so, the physician was very distraught but had no alternative but to listen as I explained what happened.

The next call I made was to my nurse manager, who had gone home for the day. She could hear the distress in my voice as I explained to her what had happened.

"How is the patient doing," she asked calmly. "Have you communicated with the physician?"

"We are monitoring the patient," I responded. "He seems okay right now, and yes, I have spoken with the doctor."

She offered reassurance, thanked me for calling her, and assured me that she would follow up the next day.

The LPN and I did communicate about what happened, but ultimately, I had to bite the bullet because even though her intentions were good to help me while I was busy assuming other duties, it was my responsibility to administer a drug in this category, not hers. I believe wholeheartedly until this day that she meant well but fell prey to being rushed and hurried and incorrectly set the pump at the incorrect rate.

Of course, I didn't get any sleep that night. I prayed that the patient would be okay and not endure harm or suffering as a result of my not following the policy that I should have hung the Integrilin instead of the LPN.

Fortunately, the patient did not suffer any adverse reaction and was discharged when I arrived to work the next day.

Several factors can cause a near-miss incident in a hospital setting. Medication errors are one of the leading causes of injury in a hospital setting. While safe medication administration is one of the essential nursing tasks we learn in school and during orientation, it is not the lack of knowledge for this critical task that leads to medication errors. Despite advances in technology, medication errors continue to occur in healthcare institutions.

Why does this continue to happen?

As mentioned in the previous chapter, external factors play a significant role that can lead to medication errors. These external factors include noisy work environments, multi-tasking, not following hospital policy (such as taking shortcuts to administer medications), and most importantly, lacking understanding of your role as an RN as it relates to delegating assignments.

Many interruptions occur during medication administration: phone calls, patients, coworkers, physicians, and visitors interrupt this important work task.

While their concerns and the need for interruption are oftentimes valid, the interruption has occurred and has shifted your focus to something else that potentially can lead to a medication error.

Effective communication with your coworkers or delegating can minimize interruptions during this critical task. Just one short cut, by attempting to bypass procedures outlined by your facility to administer medication, is a serious offense and one that will surely lead to medication errors.

In many facilities, patients wear barcoded armbands. This is a safeguard to prevent errors in medication administration. Always scan your patient's armband. Never bypass by placing other identifiers such as medical record numbers, social security numbers, or any other form of identification. This is against hospital policy and again will surely at some point cause a medication error.

Being an "old school" nurse, I still rely on the "5 rights of medication administration," which are:

1. The right patient
2. The right drug
3. The right dose
4. The right route
5. The right time

Although technology is in place, relying on the "5 rights administration" is a safe way to administer medication. Always having the patient state his or her full name while checking it against the armband is another safe practice to ensure the administration of medications. The wrong armband could have been placed on the patient, and the computer doesn't know. The computer just scans the armband.

Human error is a huge factor in medication error. Always question orders, including medications that are unclear to the physician and/or pharmacist.

Other causes of near-miss events are inadequate staffing ratios and insufficient amounts of experienced nurses delivering care to patients with multiple disease processes.

I can remember when shortly after graduating from nursing school, patients were admitted to the hospital for such routine diagnoses as a headache.

Those days are gone.

Patients who are admitted into the hospital nowadays are very ill and require nurses who are skilled and knowledgeable. That's why, as I mentioned earlier, it is critical for patient safety to *Work Smarter, Not Harder*, by adhering to the principles outlined in this guide.

Your feelings after a near-miss will be that of fear for your patient's safety, fear of personal consequences, and fear of disbelief and professional failure.

A near-miss event will always result in a root cause analysis. A root cause analysis is an investigation or an in-depth analysis of what happened in order to reveal the factors that led to the incident. What caused it to happen, and what measures can be taken to prevent it from happening in the future?

A root cause analysis team is composed of members set forth by the hospital administration. The most important thing during a root cause analysis meeting is to be honest and to analyze what happened, how it happened, how it could have been prevented, and resolutions to the problem.

Be very honest about the situation.

For me, the inability to stop and concentrate due to interruptions was my reasoning for the error on my part. It was a lack of judgment that could have had a more severe outcome.

A root analysis meeting is not a punishment session; it is a meeting to get to the root of a problem.

First and foremost, be honest about the situation if you are ever involved in a near-miss or, God forbid, a sentinel event where death has occurred as a result of your nursing judgment.

I can only imagine how it would feel to be part of a sentinel event and to live with the regret and remorse that, though unintentional, I caused the death of an individual. Your nursing career as you know it no longer exists, coupled with your living with the regret and remorse that, though unintentionally, you caused the death of an individual.

Errors in nursing can cause permanent damage, prolonged hospital stays, and death.

Nursing is an interdisciplinary profession, meaning working collaboratively with other members of the health care team with mutual respect, teamwork, and communication to achieve safe patient outcomes and to prevent near miss and sentinel events.

Knowing your job responsibilities and the job duties of personnel under your jurisdiction is a vital part of *working smarter, not harder*.

Consider this:

What are some areas of improvement you can make on your unit to prevent near miss or sentinel events? Have you ever experienced a 'near-miss' or a sentinel event in your career? What was the outcome, and what have you done differently to prevent its reoccurrence?

Work Smarter, Not Harder

CHAPTER SIX
Workplace Bullying and Violence

You cannot work smarter in any job until you learn how to manage workplace bullying and lateral violence. The same applies to the field of healthcare.

I can remember when my twin sister and I lived in Chicago before my mother became ill. We were constantly confronted by a neighbor who lived a few doors away from us. Every day, my sister and I looked forward to the ice cream truck to enjoy a double-dipped chocolate ice cream cone. Every day, this girl, who I will call Jackie, would come and for no reason at all, just knock over our ice cream. We were probably six or seven-years-old at the time.

Jackie was probably ten or eleven-years-old, clearly bigger and older than we were. We would just cry and wonder what we had done to deserve this. We were from the south, where people got along and had never been confronted or exposed to this type of behavior.

The two of us together could not fight her.

"If you tell it," Jackie hissed, "I'm going to have my brothers jump on you!"

Jackie was mean and cruel to us every day. It got to the point that my sister and I didn't enjoy going out to play anymore. Our mother quickly noticed something was wrong.

Once our mother got to the bottom of what was going on, Jackie and her brothers never bothered us again.

Being bullied leaves you fearful with a feeling of helplessness that cannot be described. The intent of the person who is doing the bullying is to instill fear in order to elicit control over the person or persons being bullied. This is a prominent problem in nursing and prevalent in all settings.

Workplace bullying can be defined as rude, repeated, and disrespectful actions and words intended to offend, humiliate, and distress others in the workplace. I was shocked when I experienced this type of behavior. I could not believe, with the seriousness of our occupation, this type of behavior existed or was tolerated.

In my younger years of nursing, I was assigned the worst patients on the floor. It seems like I always got the first admission, and no one ever offered to help. I didn't ask for help either. I probably wanted to show them that "I could do it myself." Struggling to complete my tasks, I listened as some of my coworkers sat around the nurse's station, laughing and talking about non-work-related conversations. It was as if they wanted to see how long or how much I could take (or at least, this is how I felt). Because I was young, I didn't know how to speak up for myself, and honestly, I felt intimidated by the older, more experienced nurses with titles.

Lateral violence or violence between coworkers causes nurse burnout, feelings of low self-esteem, and increased absenteeism. Lateral violence can be between certain groups of the healthcare team.

I have witnessed this type of violence in the workplace where certain groups feel as if they are superior, perpetuate an "us" vs. "them" mentality, or simply refuse to perform their respective job duties.

I have overheard conversations involving "getting your car keyed" or phrases such as "snitches get stitches."

Every employee, regardless of where employed, has the right to be treated with respect and the right to express his or her feelings and concerns as it relates to patient care and safety.

I personally know nurses who have had their nice cars "keyed."

How can you tolerate or work in an environment where these types of behaviors are the acceptable norm?

First, communicate your concerns with your nurse manager. Continue to perform your job duties in a professional, skillful manner, and ignore the behavior.

Stand tall, remain firm in your professional and workplace ethics, and most importantly, don't cave into these behaviors.

You can turn aggression into respect.

Hospitals are required to promote a safe work environment for their employees and have now implemented a zero-tolerance for these types of behaviors.

The implementation of reporting systems to report these types of behaviors is available in some hospital facilities.

Most of all, do not conform to these behaviors, which is exactly what bullies want you to do. With every new nurse that comes, this pattern of behavior is recognized, and soon new nurses will be socialized into this negative practice.

Work smarter, not harder, by not conforming to these negative practices.

Consider this:

Have you ever identified or experienced workplace bullying or violence? If so, how did you manage it?

Work Smarter, Not Harder

Work Smarter, Not Harder

CHAPTER SEVEN
Communication is Key

Another essential and critical component of *Working Smarter, Not Harder* is learning how to attain and maintain effective interpersonal communication with coworkers, nurse managers, physicians, and other administrative staff.

I cannot overemphasize the importance of effective communication in nursing. Because ineffective communication is the cornerstone for so many areas of default, I will spend a little more time on this topic.

Communication, verbal and non-verbal, among members of the health care team, can heal or destroy us as individuals, cause cultural divides, and create misunderstandings that will lead to ineffective outcomes. Moreover, poor communication can result in workplace stress, low morale, poor job performance, burnout, and high nurse turnover, just to name a few.

Workplace safety, lateral violence, and bullying are issues that affect nursing today more than ever before, with the culprit being that of ineffective communication.

No doubt, throughout your nursing career and life, there will be conflicts that can lead to ineffective communication resulting in feelings of frustration, anger, and doubt. Subsequently, these feelings can lead to poor job performance, uncooperative efforts, poor or loss of team spirit, and wasting of invaluable amounts of time, time that can be spent building positive, valuable work experiences.

Consider the following potential pitfalls:

- **Cultural Diversity**: Nursing is becoming more and more culturally diverse. With this being said, I can't stress enough the importance of getting to know your coworker's cultural beliefs, behaviors, and practices. Learning to respect each other's differences and valuing those differences will invite a level of trust built on mutual respect.

- **Poor Conflict Resolution and Management**: It is okay to disagree. We are all adults, and sometimes there will be situations that can't be avoided. Try to remain calm and don't draw negative conclusions until you've had the opportunity to communicate when emotions are not running high. Use face-to-face communication rather than digital communication. Electronic communication can be damaging when intentions are misunderstood. Communicating in person allows for questions and clarification. Know your chain of command when communicating concerns or conflicts. Oftentimes, conflicts can be resolved on a "local level."

- **Inability to Set Boundaries**: Learn how to say, "No," or "I don't feel comfortable performing this task at this time," or "Please, may I observe you as I've only performed this task a few times." Do not agree to perform any duties outside of your scope of practice or to allow anyone under your jurisdiction to perform job functions that are clearly your responsibility (just as I learned from the near-miss incident described earlier). You can say "No" in a professional manner. This will relay to the individual that you're not "refusing" to perform a task but are instead "emphasizing" your abilities (or lack thereof). Communicate further learning needs or objectives with your clinical preceptor, nursing educator, and nurse manager.

- **Poor Self-image or Self-esteem**: As a new graduate, I can truly relate to the lack of confidence and knowledge in comparison to others (Being overly confident can also cause one not to ask for help when needed, which is equally as dangerous). A lack of confidence (or knowledge) is a feeling that is typical for new graduates, but I promise it will dissipate. When your knowledge base broadens, your confidence will begin to soar!

My particular area of low self-esteem was evidenced when as a new nurse, I encountered a surgical team making rounds. They entered the patient's room while I was performing a task and as if I were *Casper the Friendly Ghost*, they never acknowledged my presence and immediately took over the conversation that I was engaged in with my patient. They didn't bother to ask me if it was okay to interrupt my conversation or work. I would have gladly stepped aside as I understood the importance of their time. Instead of speaking about my concerns, I internalized my feelings.

My suggestion is that you do not allow or tolerate this type of behavior.

In a professional manner (and not in front of the patient), kindly say, "I would appreciate next time …" If the behavior continues, talk to your nurse manager about how to handle these types of situations.

Sometimes problems have to be addressed on higher levels. Remember, nursing is an interdisciplinary profession, and everyone should be treated with a professional level of respect.

Keep in mind and learn, as I have, what battles to fight. Some are just not worth it. Know which ones are and pursue them first by talking to someone who will advise properly how to handle such situations.

I'm more seasoned now, so I've learned to step back and just simply listen. Everything does not require a response or feedback unless asked.

Most importantly, don't internalize stress or perceived perceptions.

- **Workplace Gossip**: This is a no-no, hands down! I have experienced and regretfully but honestly engaged in this type of behavior. I can tell you from experience that this behavior wreaks havoc on the job. Participating in gossip demonstrates a lack of integrity and honesty. Own up to your mistakes, and if anyone brings gossip to you, I will pass on the advice my grandmother gave to me: "A dog that brings a bone carries a bone." Dismiss the gossip by excusing yourself or changing the conversation.

If that doesn't work for the hardcore gossipers, simply and kindly say, "I don't care to be involved in this conversation," and remove yourself from the scene. Seems cold? It may be, but you'll be glad that you didn't involve yourself. Find something productive to do instead.

- **Confidentiality**: Failing to report pertinent information or "No Talk" is delicate. The rules for reporting such information is delicate at best. "No Talk" issues can result in serious consequences such as patient harm or, in extreme cases, death.

One such "No Talk" reason would be witnessing a nurse impaired due to alcohol or drug ingestion.

One of the main reasons nurses "don't talk" is due to fear, fear of retaliation, fear of rejection, etc. from other coworkers.

Confidentiality in the workplace is crucial in these types of situations. Do not assume, approach, or pass judgment on the individual in question. Instead, observe the behavior while maintaining the observations in writing and keeping it confidential.

Approach your nurse manager confidentially with your observations. It will be left up to his or her discretion to make any decisions regarding the situation. If you don't report the situation, you are driving the getaway car and, in essence, condoning an unethical behavior.

Consider this:

How can you improve communication? Are you able to communicate effectively on the job?

CHAPTER EIGHT
Prioritizing Patient Care

Now that we've hit some of the key areas in *working smarter, not harder*, it's time to focus on another key element in your nursing journey.

Prioritizing patient care, including time management, is vital to your success as a nurse. Before we talk about prioritizing patient care, it is important for me to share with you that before you can take care of anyone, including your family, you must take care of yourself first.

Place priority on yourself first, then and only then will you be able to manage and prioritize care for your patients effectively.

Taking care of yourself includes spending quiet time in meditation, physical exercise, and healthy eating. These behaviors will reduce stress and increase your energy level, which will aid in effectively taking care of your patients.

With so many tasks waiting for you as soon as you arrive to work, how do you prioritize? What do you do first?

Arrive to Work Early

First, arrive to work early to avoid being rushed and hurried. This will allow time for you to put your things away, take a deep breath, and get ready for report.

Feeling rushed and hurried at the beginning of the shift sets the tone for the remainder of the shift, and you will feel like you're playing "catch up" during the remainder of the day.

Your coworkers who have worked their shifts are ready to wind it down and prepare to go home, just as you will be when it's time for your shift to end.

Being late will disrupt the workflow of your unit. There could be occasions where emergencies will arise, and you might have to be late, but please address these concerns with your manager. A continued pattern of tardiness reflects disrespect for your place of employment, and you may be subject to disciplinary actions. Arrive to work early, ready to begin your shift.

Assess the Day

I strongly advocate walking rounds as a part of prioritizing patient care. Walking rounds is a safe, interactive handoff that allows the opportunity for questions, up-to-date information, and most importantly, a visual inspection of the patient before you assume care.

If there are issues, they can be handled at this point.

A quick assessment of your patients during walking rounds will give you an idea of how to prioritize care for the shift. Some unit policies require walking rounds. This practice waxes and wanes at times, but do not assume care for anyone you have not laid eyes on.

If you do assume care for a patient without walking rounds, when you walk in the room and find a problem, it's yours. It will throw you off your routine.

Please understand that a patient's condition can change from minute to minute, and walking rounds establishes a baseline for your initial assessment. Walking rounds is a safe practice as well as a priority.

Every nurse has his or her own routine.

My routine will be different from yours and vice versa. You will develop your own system and routine for managing your patient load after orientation.

After reporting, if there is nothing that requires my immediate attention, I begin to prepare my medication cart with supplies that may be low (i.e., medicine cups, alcohol prep pads, syringes, supplies for checking blood glucose, etc.).

A pet-peeve of mine is coming on to a shift and finding the medication cart unstocked. I know at the end of your shift, you're exhausted and ready to leave, but it only takes a minute to restock. This small task adds valuable time for the oncoming nurse.

Restocking your medication cart minimizes walking to get items that you could have had in the first place.

This practice saves time and is more efficient. Preparation is a valuable lesson in prioritizing patient care.

These really are huge time savers and will certainly be appreciated by the nurse following you.

Manage Time Wisely

Time management, another part of *working smarter, not harder*, is the ability to get tasks accomplished in a timely, professional, and most importantly, safe manner.

Determine which patients require your immediate attention and those patients who may require a little longer time for nursing care.

There is no magic formula for this as each patient's needs are different, and with time, you will gain a feel for what tasks are needed right away or can be staggered into your shift time.

Make your rounds immediately for your patient assessment, medication administration, and nursing documentation.

Minimize distractions by not falling into conversations that will distract you from the task at hand. There will always be interruptions along the way, such as phone calls from physicians or labs to report critical lab alerts, etc.

Complete tasks promptly while always maintaining safety. This is to allow for extra time in the event that one of your patients worsens and requires extra attention and time from you.

Stay organized by knowing your patient's condition, history, and current vital signs or other pertinent information should a physician call and need a quick update.

Computers have helped a lot in staying organized, but from time to time, we still need to write, as in report.

Learn to delegate tasks and seek out and ask for help if needed. Know the job responsibilities of other ancillary staff and their job duties, such as nursing assistants who are certified to perform tasks and can take some of the load from you.

Utilize your resources to the fullest. Many facilities have PICC teams. A PICC team is a group of nurses who are specialized in attaining peripheral IV access. Why waste time sticking a patient when you have a team of skilled nurses with advanced equipment who can quickly access a patient's veins?

This not only saves you time but also saves the patient from being stuck multiple times.

Be a Team Player. Lend a helping hand. When a coworker is drowning, throw in a life jacket. One thing to know about nursing is it could be "their" day today and "yours" tomorrow. You would want someone to help you. Ask if you can help pass out meds if coworkers are behind schedule or perform some other task to help them get through.

Take Breaks. Factor in time to take your breaks. This is one of the downfalls of nursing, not breaking and not eating. I have witnessed nurses who have almost passed out trying to get finished by foregoing their break time. This is a habit that you should not begin.

How can you effectively take care of someone when your judgment is clouded due to hypoglycemia?

Granted, there are times when you will not have time to eat, drink, or even go to the restroom. As a backup, always keep a healthy protein snack in your locker or pocket for those times when a break may not be timely.

People, who aren't nurses will ask, "How is it that you don't get a break?"

> *Remember the cartoon, The Flintstones? When the whistle blew, Fred grabbed his lunch pail and off he went. No, nursing does not operate this way.*

It's not that we don't want a break, but nursing is not working on an assembly line. The job must be completed. We can't carry it home or come back the next day and pick up where we left off. Medications must be administered, procedures must be completed, and most importantly, documentation must be completed. If a patient worsens and your documentation is not done or lacking vital information, you have left yourself wide open for litigation.

Learn to slow down. Nurses run marathons. We have so many tasks to complete within a certain timeframe. It is important to slow down to avoid potentially dangerous outcomes for our patients and ourselves.

Thank God for needless syringes!

The risk of needle puncture incidents has declined but is still a huge problem in our profession. Protect yourself by slowing down.

I worked with a nurse who unfortunately had a needle stick from an HIV positive patient, acquired HIV-AIDS, and is now deceased.

How tragic!

Protect yourself from blood/body fluid splashes and sticks by always following hospital policy and wearing the appropriate PPE's (Personal Protective Equipment). If someone is rushing you to draw blood and you feel pressured by time, please stop, take a deep breath, and only complete the task when you feel that you can focus on the task at hand.

Survey the day. At the end of your shift, always reevaluate, analyze, and ask, "How or what could I have done differently to make the day better or less hectic?"

Remember, no two days are alike; some days will be good, and others will be terrible. But always keep in mind that the shift will end and focus on keeping your patients safe while under your care.

Nursing school provides the theory and clinical foundation for a successful nursing path. However, the real learning begins when you graduate, pass the state board, and begin to practice on your own license.

You realize that nursing is your livelihood, and to maintain an unrestricted nursing license is something that will take hard work in order to *Work Smarter, Not Harder.*

Some lessons in nursing are not learned in nursing school.

You begin to acquire innate or "gut feelings" when something is not right. You will learn this as you mature along your journey.

Learn to listen to your "gut feelings" and instincts. Communicate any concerns along the way, and become familiar with your patients, paying close attention to trends or changes from their baselines.

Consider this:

Name three behaviors that you can modify or initiate to prioritize patient care. Are you taking time for yourself, managing stress? If not, what's preventing you from doing so?

Work Smarter, Not Harder

CHAPTER NINE
Learn to Listen

Above all, learn to listen!

I can recall that one of the prerequisite courses for nursing was music appreciation. I thought to myself, "What does music have to do with nursing?"

After starting the class, it became one of my favorite subjects. What I learned is that we don't listen as well as we think. My instructor would take pieces of music from Beethoven, Mozart, and other music scholars, and we had to identify the piece, even if it was started in the middle. That meant we had to listen very intensely to identify the music. I would wear headphones and listen very carefully to the pieces of music, learning to identify the different musical notes, changes in tempo, etc.

Sometimes, we have the habit of just listening to part of a conversation, so intent on thinking about what our response will be that we miss out on the whole conversation. Ineffective communication (including failing to listen) leads to a breakdown in understanding and often leads to miscommunication and subsequent errors in nursing care.

Practice repeating what someone said to you in terms like, "Did I understand you to say ..." or "I didn't understand what you said. Can you please repeat that in a way I can understand?"

Asking for clarification puts you ahead of the listening game. Never assume what you thought someone said; make sure you know what he or she said. This is extremely important when communicating with physicians, for example taking telephone orders.

Due to electronic ordering, telephone orders are almost obsolete, but in some cases, this may be the only way to take a physician's order. Always repeat the order back to the physician, asking for clarification if the order is unclear or lacks full instructions. Obtain the physician's full name (you'd be surprised by the number of doctors with the same last name in a hospital). Most importantly, ensure correct patient identification per your hospital policy.

I'm so glad I listened to a patient who was under my care this particular day.

"I'm not gonna make it," the [cardiac patient] said weakly to me. "Can you call my wife for me?"

We had recognized a change in his condition and called a rapid response team (RRT) to assist him.

Everyone around him, including me, was busy, rushing to perform the needed tasks.

Instead of responding, "Oh, let's wait; you'll get better. We'll call later." I listened to him (as well as my *gut feelings*) and called the patient's wife.

Handing him the phone, he spoke softly into the receiver, "I need you to come now. I don't think I'm gonna make it," he repeated.

My heart went out to him as I took the phone from him and hung it up.

While we had seen a slight improvement in his condition, he was still not out of the woods.

The patient's wife arrived with other family members, including his grandchildren. They spent time with him as we continued to stabilize him.

Long story short, his condition required transferring him to ICU. My shift ended, but when I returned to work the next day, I learned that he had passed.

I'm so thankful that I listened to him and let him speak to this wife. That was the last time he saw his wife and family.

Sometimes things that we brush off as small really do have very significant consequences.

Imagine being the person in the hospital bed. Imagine the person being someone whom you loved dearly. Literally, place yourself in your mind's eye for a while as that person lying in bed. Practice it sometimes. You will feel differently. You would never be rude or unkind to yourself or someone you love, would you?

I have been on the other side of the bed twice, and every time I experienced it, it was a very helpless feeling. Depending on someone else to care for you is a very humbling experience.

When I was in labor with my first son, I was in so much pain. Pain like that freezes time. I know the nurse had probably just told me she was going to get my pain meds, but because the pain was so intense, it seemed like an hour!

I kept hitting the call light like a crazy woman, and I'm sure the nurse was saying to herself, "God, why does she keep calling? I just told her a minute ago I'd be there."

It's funny now when I think back on it, but the pain was real. Try thinking about your own personal experiences when dealing with difficult patients. It will help you walk a mile in that person's shoes.

Consider this:

Are you a good listener? Do you listen to your "gut feelings?" How can you improve your listening skills?

_____

_____

_____

_____

_____

_____

_____

_____

_____

THE DIRTY DOZEN
Twelve Pitfalls to Workplace Success

I worked for the airline industry for almost ten years as a Customer Service Agent. The Federal Aviation Administration (FAA) has identified twelve common mistakes made in the aviation workplace. I find these mistakes can apply to nearly every area of occupation:

1. *Lack of Communication* (failure to transmit, receive, or provide enough information to complete a task) – Never assume anything. Only 30 percent of verbal communication is received and understood by either side of a conversation.

2. *Complacency* (overconfidence based on repeated experience performing tasks) – Avoid the tendency to see what you expect to see.

3. *Lack of Knowledge* (lack of understanding your job role, training, procedures, etc.) – Don't' guess. Know or ask when you don't know. Participate in training.

4. *Distractions* (anything that draws your attention away from the task at hand) – Stay focused on one task at a time.

5. *Lack of Teamwork* (failure to work together to complete a shared goal) – Build a solid team. Discuss how tasks should be done.

6. *Fatigue* (physical and/or mental exhaustion that threatens work performance) – Balance work and home, providing time for rest, family, exercise, and other stress-reducing activities.

7. *Lack of Resources* (not having enough people, equipment, time, etc. to complete a task) – Communicate your needs or concerns to your nurse manager, not to coworkers who can do no more than you.

8. *Pressure* (real or perceived forces demanding high-level job performance) – Communicate concerns. Ask for extra help.

9. *Lack of Assertiveness* (failure to speak up or document concerns and instructions, orders, or actions of others) – Express your feelings, opinions, beliefs, and needs in a positive, productive manner.

10. *Stress* (a physical or emotional factor that causes physical or mental tension) – Manage stress before it happens. Listen to your body, seek help, take short breaks, and exercise.

11. *Lack of Awareness* (failure to recognize a situation, to understand what it is, and to predict the outcome) – Fully understand policies, procedures, and your job responsibilities.

12. *Norms* (expected, yet unwritten rules of behaviors) – Existing norms don't make procedures right. Identify negative norms. When in doubt, defer to your facility policy and procedures.

Consider this:

How many "dirty dozens" are you dealing with on your job? What changes are you willing to make?

CONCLUSION
An Art of the Heart

Nursing is not a scripted occupation. No two days are alike. Some days, there are happy endings, and others end sadly. But to each day brings a new lesson that brings you closer to being that nurse who is highly professional, skilled, knowledgeable, and above all, knows how to *Work Smarter, Not Harder.*

Know that you are valued and respected.

Let me repeat that:

Know that you are valued and respected.

We should be proud and have a level of confidence assuring our patients that they are in good hands. We stand between life and death for our patients.

When I realized and understood that concept, my perception of nursing changed.

There were many days when I would leave my unit for the day with second thoughts about coming back to work. I entertained the idea of leaving the profession entirely.

Seriously, you will have days like that.

Likely, many of you have felt like, "I can't do this anymore."

My feet would hurt so badly that I didn't' think I could take another step. But then I'd think about the huge impact and the awesome responsibility that I have on my patients, coworkers, and the nursing profession. Still, I came back.

And for 30+ years now, I've kept coming back.

Nurses see things that doctors don't see. We are the 24-hour, around-the-clock watchful eyes that carefully monitor and observe. Our intuition tells us when a problem begins to raise its ugly head.

We know that time is valuable, so we don't waste it.

As they say in the cardiac unit, "Time is a muscle."

For every minute we waste on a person having a heart attack, it cost cardiac muscle that will have a major impact on the outcome and quality of their life.

We don't wait; we respond.

When I look back over my career, I wouldn't change a thing. My career has shaped me into the proud, professional nurse I am today – mistakes and all.

Thankfully, with God's blessings, no serious harm occurred to any patient under my care.

No bragging rights, just simply following the training, policies, and tips others shared with me. By following the advice that I've shared with you, you too can have a successful career in nursing.

Always imagine yourself being that patient in the bed, and care for them as if they were you or a loved one.

Remember, *Work Smarter, Not Harder.*

Nursing really is an art of the heart.

ABOUT THE AUTHOR

Joann Coleman, a professional Registered Nurse, mentor, and preceptor, has over 30 years of nursing experience. In addition to mentoring and teaching graduate nurses, she possesses a broad skill set and theoretical knowledge base in nursing.

The author's passion for molding and mentoring nurses is what motivates and inspires her each day.

Joann grew up in a small rural town in Arkansas before moving to Chicago.

She now resides in Memphis, TN, with her husband.